BOOST YOUR BRAINPOWER
A GUIDE TO IMPROVING YOUR MEMORY & FOCUS

Dr. Eric Kaplan, DC, FACFN

Contents

Introduction

My interest in health started when I was thirteen years old. I was a very sick child. I had bad acne, low energy, and, worst of all, I was overweight. Actually, according to the World Health Organization and my pediatrician, I was obese. In addition, every morning I started my day coughing up thick phlegm from chronic bronchitis—largely due to the fact that I was exposed to second-hand cigarette smoke at home. To top it off, I had terrible "brain fog," which affected my academic and sports performance due to lack of focus, organization, planning, and motivation.

When my mother asked the doctor what we should do, his solution was that I should take antibiotics and steroids. Growing up in the 1980s, nobody ever questioned the doctor, so of course, I had to take the medications. However, the prescriptions made me super sick. I was constantly nauseous and dizzy, and I vomited over ten times a day because of these harmful medications. Since I was embarrassed about always throwing up, I stopped going outside to play with my friends. I became depressed, and I felt hopeless. If I was doing what the doctor said and feeling even worse, I realized, I might have to live like this for the rest of my life.

I was desperate to find a solution. Luckily, I didn't even have to leave my own house to find it. My father, Dr. Larry Kaplan, changed my life forever by introducing me to the Natural Hygiene Society. Once I showed a deep interest in health and well-being, he began paying for all my health seminars and education, buying me all the health books I could imagine, purchasing very healthy food, and leading me in the right direction.

One of the first things I learned from the Natural Hygiene Society was that dairy is a major cause of congestion in the lungs. I made the connection that quitting dairy might help my chronic bronchitis. As a result, I eliminated all dairy from my diet. That meant no cheese, milk, yogurt, ranch dressing, creamy sauces, butter, and—do I dare say it—no ice cream! Because I was so sick and tired of being sick and tired, I decided to give it a try. To my amazement, within one month of quitting dairy, my bronchitis was completely gone. Imagine the look on the doctor's face when I went back and told him, "Thank you, but I don't need these antibiotics or steroids anymore. I cured my bronchitis myself." Even living in the same house as a smoker, I was still able to heal myself of bronchitis just by changing my diet. This is when I first realized that food is the original and most important medicine. As Hippocrates said, "Let thy food be thy medicine and thy medicine be thy food."

Because I was only 13 years old and had treated my bronchitis with better results than my pediatrician, I became empowered. I determined that my purpose on this Earth was to be a part of the HEALTHCARE solution and not a part of the modern American "SICKCARE" problem. Consequently, as a young teenager, I decided that I wanted to become a doctor and help other people get healthy and happy. I always knew that I was going to be a different type of doctor. I pledged to focus on healing people from a holistic and integrative approach to health. Instead of taking medications and antibiotics for every condition, I realized that by altering your environment, you can eliminate almost any medical diagnosis, such as heart disease, cancer, diabetes, and even Alzheimer's disease. I began to understand that the body has an amazing potential for self-healing, as long as we give it the essentials for health and well-being.

Most people know that the modern medical community in the United States is focused on drugs and surgery. I don't blame the doctors for this. It's not their fault. I blame their education. American doctors are taught to diagnose a condition and then prescribe the medication that treats that disease. This approach started many years ago when many educational institutions were funded by John D. Rockefeller, an industrialist who gave millions of dollars to medical research and development in his lifetime. Before Rockefeller was involved in the pharmaceutical industry, the medical school curriculum looked very different. Nutrition and exercise were of the utmost importance. Unfortunately, Rockefeller, being a businessman, realized that there was real money to be made in the production of drugs, so he started funding institutions that prioritized pharmacology over preventative medicine as the primary way of treating disease. A drug may only cost a penny to make, but the company that creates it can charge you a hundred dollars to purchase it. This fact changed the trajectory of medicine, and today, doctors have been brainwashed by the pharmaceutical industry to think that medicine is the only way to help with certain diseases. These companies even go as far as trying to blemish the licenses and reputations of doctors who do not promote medicine as the primary source of treatment. Since Rockefeller, education in medical schools in the United States has been focused on developing medicines to treat the symptoms of different diseases instead of getting to the root cause of the disease.

Luckily, this history is getting revealed. Medicine is just a Band-Aid for most conditions. Please do not be mistaken: if you are in an emergency, modern medicine is fantastic! If you're having a stroke, it is absolutely necessary to get to the hospital immediately, where doctors will administer the proper medication to prevent loss of blood flow to the brain or even death. If you're poisoned or having an allergic reaction, you must get to the hospital for urgent treatment. For emergencies, American medicine is great; in fact, it's the best in the world. However, the US actually ranks very low for disease prevention and chronic illnesses.

Instead of just giving in to the idea that we are helpless when it comes to our health, that we should just wait for symptoms and diseases to progress to the point where we need medications to live, we need to start from the ground up to promote a healthier society. We cannot treat our bodies carelessly and expect our health to thrive. We certainly cannot live like the average American if we expect to live a long, healthy, active, disease-free life. Most people overlook the fact that you have opportunities to heal yourself several times a day. This book will cover most of the strategies and techniques to help you do so. After reading this book, however, you must take action! Do not wait until Monday. Take action immediately. The best decision I ever made after my first seminar was to take immediate action and avoid putting it off until tomorrow.

When I was thirteen, I took immediate action by changing my diet. I quit dairy and became a vegan. However, it wasn't becoming vegan that made me healthy. It was that I had stopped eating fish containing mercury, cows injected with steroids, turkeys injected with antibiotics, chickens stuck in small cages and fed GMO corn, candy and soda filled with processed sugar, deli meats containing preservatives, Gatorade with food dyes, milk from stressed-out cows, and foods containing pesticides, herbicides, artificial flavors, and other toxic chemicals. Being vegan doesn't automatically make you healthy. There are many "junk food vegans and vegetarians" that are just as sick as omnivores. If you eat a lot of processed food, sugar, bread products, and pasta, or food loaded with dyes and preservatives, you cannot expect to be healthy. Humans need to eat natural foods from the earth like they did thousands of years ago, keeping their diet balanced, seasonal, and fresh.

In high school, I became one of the healthy vegans. I didn't eat any sugar or candy—I lived off of fruit, vegetables, beans, nuts, and seeds. My fellow students would call me "Nuts and Berries" and teased me because of the way I ate, but I didn't care, because changing my diet had countless benefits almost immediately. I lost tons of body fat, my skin cleared up, my bronchitis was cured, my energy improved, and even my sports performance enhanced. I started growing taller and had more confidence. I began doing better in school and getting into honors classes. Girls started talking to me more. I grew much happier and healthier. My life completely changed in amazing ways, and I felt that I needed to share this with the world. I can guarantee that if you change your diet strictly and dramatically, and focus on eating reasonable portions of fresh food, your body and your life will change rather quickly.

In this book, we will not only review how nutrition can be used to improve brain function, but how sixteen other easy, magical habits will keep you living a long, healthy, high-quality life.

The reason I am so passionate about high quality of life stems from my experience with my Grandma Dottie. When I was a young child, my grandmother and I used to spend a lot of time together since she lived in Brooklyn, and I lived not too far away in New Jersey. But after she moved to Florida, I saw her less frequently. Sadly, I became more aware of her diminishing health with each visit. When she moved to Florida, she stopped doing all the things that were keeping her healthy. In Brooklyn, she did lots of activities—she played tennis, went dancing, played cards with her friends, and was always out socializing. She was also a great cook, and she kept her house immaculate. She had a very active social life, spending time with family and friends. She took great pride in her appearance, always looking so elegant and classy.

After her years in Florida, I sensed something had changed with Grandma Dottie. The first things I noticed were little incidents like her opening the refrigerator door and forgetting what she wanted. She started forgetting where she put her keys. She had always been good at remembering people's names, but after a few years in Florida, forgetting people's names became a lot more frequent.

Please understand that this does not mean that if you ever lost your keys or forgot someone's name that you have Alzheimer's. But what it does mean is that you should not just accept that these things happen as you get older. If you follow the guidelines in this book, you may be able to prevent memory and focus problems. Remember that my grandma's Alzheimer's didn't develop in a few months in Florida; it happened over years and years. The good news is that because it takes years and years to develop, we can detect early warning signs of Alzheimer's disease and prevent it. For example, loss of sense of smell can occur 40 years before any memory loss, so it is vital to get your sense of smell checked immediately. In addition to a smell test, I suggest taking the written Montreal Cognitive Assessment test— which can be downloaded for free—to see if you are at risk as well. A normal score is at least 26 points out of the possible 30.

The ideal approach, however, is to actually prevent Alzheimer's from developing in the first place. Neuroscience and functional neurology researchers have found there are lots of different ways to reverse Alzheimer's and dementia. This book will teach you the changes you can make to your lifestyle to start the process of reversing it and show you how to boost your brainpower so you can prevent future problems as well.

Getting back to my Grandma Dottie: as her brain deteriorated, I also noticed she stopped caring about how she looked and how the house looked. There was a lot more dust, and the beds weren't as neat and crisp as they used to be. Even as a fourteen-year-old, I noticed these changes. I didn't know it was Alzheimer's disease until later, when I began studying neuroscience. Before that, though, I witnessed my grandma suffer for way too many years. She lost her appetite, started losing weight, became angrier, had to wear a diaper, needed someone to bathe her because she couldn't do it herself, and eventually needed a wheelchair. She was miserable and had a poor quality of life. The worst part for me was that I would visit her, and she wouldn't even know who I was anymore. These visits were so shocking and upsetting for me that after she passed, I strove to become an expert in the brain to figure out what caused degenerative brain diseases and prevent it from happening to other people. Luckily, I started attending functional neurology seminars with Dr. Ted Carrick, where I learned about neuroplasticity and applied neuroscience. I had a new vision then. I already knew that I wanted to use nutrition to help people prevent horrible diseases like bronchitis and irritable bowel syndrome. But my new goal was to help people like my grandmother and, more generally, to help people improve their memory. If I was going to do this, I had to take my knowledge to the next level and deeply understand the brain. I owed it to her and to the world to learn as much as possible to prevent this horrible disease.

After studying neuroscience for thousands and thousands of hours, I eventually realized that all of Grandma Dottie's suffering could have been avoided if I would have been able to give her these suggestions that I know now.

Unfortunately, she passed away before I could, but her spirit lives on and was the driving force for this book. I'm going to teach you how to change the trajectory of your life by helping you take care of your brain. I know Grandma Dottie is looking down now with a big smile on her face saying, "Good Job, Eric. I'm very proud of you." So, let's get started and work together to help you find lasting health and keep your memory functioning for many years to come!

Chapter 1: As Fit as a Fiddle

Harvard researchers recently performed a study that actually proved sitting is just as bad as smoking. Of course, I am not advising you to start smoking, but I am advising you to get off your behind and start exercising today. Most people have heard all about the benefits of exercise; when you exercise, the body releases endorphins, which make you feel great and benefit both your physical and mental health.

The best time to exercise is in the morning because that is when your testosterone and cortisol levels are highest. Morning exercise will reduce anxiety and give you more energy throughout the day. The most productive way to exercise is to do activities that you love and enjoy. If you hate running on a treadmill, it will take much more effort to convince yourself to get on the treadmill every day. You need to find something fun that will help motivate you to be consistent with your physical routine. Personally, I love to ride my bike, rollerblade, swim, and dance, as well as play basketball, tennis, and soccer. It is important to mix up your exercise routine every day to challenge your brain and body and develop different muscle groups. For example, on Monday, ride a bike; on Tuesday, power walk; on Wednesday, do some pushups or sit-ups; on Thursday, take a dance class; on Friday, go for a hike; on Saturday, go kayaking on a lake; on Sunday, take a yoga or Pilates class. The key is to find activities you like to do.

Another recommendation I often give patients is to make use of their time with their kids by combining it with their daily exercise. Having children is not an excuse to stop working out. For example, I do pushups with one of my sons sitting on top of my back and sit-ups while holding my five-year-old in my arms. If you enjoy being outside, get a running stroller or a bike with a child seat attachment and take your children with you as you exercise. Bringing them along will also instill healthy habits in the kids, and they will learn from your good example.

Gardening can be used as a way to exercise, as well. Manually sawing branches, picking up large pieces of wood, digging holes in the dirt, removing roots, moving rocks, lifting heavy bags of mulch, and squatting down to weed are all workouts! And it's not only gardening that can be a workout; every activity can be used to strengthen your body and increase daily movements. If you go shopping, you can use the bags as weights. Start doing bicep curls and shoulder lifts with your shopping bags. When you do laundry, you can use the basket to do squats. When you take out the garbage, do some lunges. These weight-resistant activities are exercises that will help your brain and, in addition, help prevent osteoporosis.

I mention these activities because the gym isn't for everyone. The solution is to find an activity you love and stick with it. Just make sure you do things that make you sweat and get your heart beating faster, and add in weight-resistant activities to get the most out of your exercise routine. Starting a real workout regimen will not just improve your general health and well-being, but it will also decrease your chances of getting Alzheimer's disease in the future and boost your brainpower by improving memory and focus.

Now, we all know that we should hold ourselves accountable for exercise; this is not rocket science. However, not everyone makes decisions that will increase movement in his or her body. I find it is much easier if someone else is holding you accountable. For example, I play in a basketball league, which means my teammates are depending on me to show up. I advise you to find an exercise partner who is dependent on you. My Grandma Dottie played tennis. She had to show up or her opponent would be very upset with her. When she went dancing, her dance partner held her accountable. If your activity is running, get a running partner. If it is biking, join a biking group. Exercising is always more likely to be sustained over the long haul if you have support, accountability, and motivation from others.

Chapter 2: You Are What You Eat

We can all agree that almost everyone knows, at least in theory, that they should eat healthy foods. People agree that eating fruits and vegetables has a multitude of benefits, like providing our bodies with whole-food sources of vitamins, minerals, fiber, and macronutrients (fats, proteins, and carbohydrates) that we need to help keep our bodies running smoothly. Eating proper nutrients helps keep our organs functioning and provides our body with the raw materials it needs to build healthy bones and produce healthy blood. It benefits digestion, metabolism, and, most importantly, the way the brain functions.

Eating bad foods, on the other hand, can harm your brain. If you consume highly inflammatory foods, your brain connections will decrease. These foods can cause a variety of problems such as trouble with memory, focus, motivation, organization, time management, depression, anxiety, anger, and aggression. The most common inflammatory foods consumed are bread, pasta, sugar, desserts, alcohol, dairy, coffee, corn, and soy products. Usually, the first medical problems that occur after consuming these foods are high cholesterol and diabetes.

Diabetes is one of the primary causes of memory loss. In fact, neuroscientists have considered changing the name of Alzheimer's disease to Diabetes Type III. When patients come to me concerned about their memory, one of the first things I teach them is the relationship between glucose levels and the homeostasis of their brain and body. After about six weeks of following the Healthy Eating Cheatsheet seen on page 15, patients start to notice a dramatic change in their blood work. I always explain to diabetic patients that adopting a strict diet and exercise routine is all they need to do to change their trajectory and get their glucose levels in their blood work within the normal range. To boost your brainpower, improve function, and reduce your risk of developing diabetes or Alzheimer's, your hemoglobin A1C levels should be under 5.7%, and fasting glucose should be under 100 mg/dL.

I remember one patient who came to me looking for help, whom we'll call Rosa. She was a Type II Diabetic taking Metformin. Rosa decided to adopt a restricted carbohydrate and sugar-free diet. Six weeks later, she actually had to be taken off of her medication by her doctor because her levels had changed so dramatically. Her doctor even said, "Pharmaceutical companies are going to go out of business. This is the cure for diabetes." But this is not the cure for diabetes; it just helps to prevent it or reverse it. The secret is that if you use diet and exercise to your advantage, your hemoglobin A1C and fasting glucose levels will be maintained, and you will feel better, function better, and live better.

The quickest and healthiest way to accomplish a dramatic change like Rosa's is to adopt a diet of mostly proteins, fats, and vegetables. Some of the healthiest foods to eat are avocados, blueberries, green and leafy vegetables, turmeric, eggs, fish, walnuts, broccoli, carrots, and coconut. I would recommend restricting oats, alcohol, dairy, bread, rice, wheat, barley, rye, oatmeal, cereal, crackers, muffins, bagels, croissants, sugar, juices, soda, and candy. After six weeks, you will notice a big difference in your blood work and reduce your chances of developing memory loss, cancer, diabetes, heart disease, and all kinds of other diseases and disorders.

When it comes to buckling down and eating healthy foods, many Americans feel like they are too busy. Of course, it is much easier to go through a drive-thru restaurant on your way home from work. More than just serving the wrong types of food, though, these restaurants pump their food with salt, fat, and sugar, which overload your senses and taste buds and make the food addictive. No matter how attractive or "healthy" the branding looks, these fast-food restaurants simply do not care about your lasting health; they only care about their profits.

We need food with high-quality nutrition, and we can't trust companies to make this food for us—so what's the solution to this unavoidable problem? For starters, I recommend learning how to cook so you can eat at home. That is not to say that everyone needs to be a five-star chef, but everyone can learn basic preparations and some simple cooking tricks. If a lack of time is the reason you do not cook, you might need to use some creative solutions like investing in a crockpot, doing meal-prep on the weekends, or even making food in advance and freezing it. To motivate yourself to cook your own food, remember that only *you* have your health's best interests in mind. Besides, starting a cooking routine might actually be fun. Many people find cooking relaxing and rewarding, but like everything else, it takes some practice and adjustment.

If you don't think you like cooking or feel you don't know how to cook, try to watch some healthy cooking shows on the internet for inspiration. The internet is an incredible source for all kinds of simple recipes. You can easily search for recipes by looking up, for example, "ketogenic salad dressings" or "easy-to-make vegetarian dinner ideas." Whatever recipes you decide on, I recommend that you plan your meals, make a list for the grocery store, and stick to that list. Make sure you're not hungry when you go grocery shopping. We really get into trouble in the grocery store when we don't have ideas for meals and we're hungry. This aimless hunger makes us more susceptible to consumer marketing and thinly veiled junk food.

Even though there's an extensive list of foods you shouldn't eat, there are plenty of foods that you can eat and still be healthy. These include fruits, vegetables, nuts, seeds, fish, eggs, poultry, and meat. To get all of your nutrients and boost your brainpower, I recommend eating at least one food for each color of the rainbow every day. I would also advise you to get all your foods organic, especially foods that have edible skin like apples, strawberries, and grapes. These fruits are typically sprayed with pesticides like Round-Up that seep into the fruit. As a result, eating these fruits can expose you to harsh chemicals that can cause a toxic overload, inflammation, and lead to neurological disorders. For animal products, buy wild fish, grass-fed beef, free-range chicken and eggs, and make sure none of the animals have been given antibiotics, hormones, or steroids.

Let eating healthy food become a habit for you. Once people understand how delicious healthy food can be, they forget about all the other food they used to eat that made them feel terrible. Having strong digestion, good brain function, and energy to do all the things you love is the real reward, so consider making a major diet change today.

HEALTHY EATING CHEATSHEET

Below is my Healthy Eating Cheatsheet. It is designed for the average American. Please keep in mind that everyone is different, and this specific plan may not apply to you if you have certain allergies or medical conditions.

FOODS TO ELIMINATE

- Alcohol
- Amaranth
- Amino peptide complex
- Artificial sweeteners
- Artificial flavors
- Avena sativa
- Barley
- Beta-glucan
- Blue cheeses
- Breaded foods
- Brown rice syrup
- Buckwheat
- Bulgur
- Butter
- Canned baked beans
- Caramel color
- Cereals
- Cheese
- Chocolate
- Chocolate milk
- Coffee
- Cold cuts
- Colloidal oatmeal
- Commercial bullion/broths
- Communion wafers
- Corn
- Couscous
- Cured meats
- Cyclodextrin
- Dairy
- Dextrin
- Dextrin palmitate

- Energy bars
- Farina
- Fermented grain extract
- Flavored coffees and teas
- Food dyes
- French fries
- Fried vegetables
- Fruit fillings and puddings
- Ghee
- Graham flour
- Gravy
- Hemp
- Hordeum distichon
- Hordeum vulgare
- Hot dogs
- Hydrolysate
- Hydrolyzed malt extract
- Hydrolyzed soy protein
- Hydrolyzed vegetable protein
- Hydrolyzed wheat protein
- Ice cream
- Imitation bacon
- Imitation crab meat
- Instant hot drinks
- Kamut matzo
- Ketchup
- Laurdimonium hydroxypropyl
- Malt/malt flavoring
- Malt extract
- Maltodextrin
- Malt vinegar
- Mayonnaise
- Meatballs
- Meatloaf
- Milk
- Millet
- Modified food starch
- Natural flavoring
- Non-dairy creamer
- Nutritional yeast
- Oats
- Peanuts
- Phytosphingosine extract
- Polish wheat
- Potato processed cheese (e.g., Velveeta)
- Rice
- Roasted nuts
- Root beer
- Rye
- Sausage
- Secale cereale
- Seitan
- Semolina
- Sesame
- Sorghum
- Soups
- Soy
- Soy sauce
- Spelt
- Stearyl dimonium hydroxypropyl
- Store-bought marinade
- Store-bought salad dressings

- Sugar/Sugar replacements
- Syrups
- Tabbouleh
- Tapioca
- Teff
- Tempura
- Teriyaki sauce
- Trail mix
- Triticale
- Triticum aestivum
- Triticum vulgare
- Vegetable protein
- Veggie burgers
- Vitamin E (Tocopherol)
- Wheat
- Wheat germ
- Wheat germ oil
- Wheatgrass
- Yeast
- Yeast extract

APPROVED FOODS TO EAT

VEGETABLES

- Anise
- Arrowroot
- Artichoke
- Arugula
- Asparagus
- Bamboo shoots
- Basil
- Bean sprouts
- Beets
- Bell pepper
- Bitter melon
- Black-eyed peas
- Bok choy
- Breadfruit
- Broccoli
- Broccolini
- Broccoli rabe
- Brussels sprouts
- Cabbage
- Cantaloupe
- Carrot
- Cauliflower
- Cayenne pepper
- Celery
- Chard/Swiss chard
- Chayote
- Cherry tomatoes
- Chicory
- Chili peppers
- Chives
- Cilantro
- Collard greens
- Cucumber
- Daikon
- Dandelion
- Dill
- Dinosaur kale/Lacinatokale
- Edamame
- Eggplant/Aubergine
- Endive
- Escarole
- Fennel
- Fiddlehead fern
- Garlic
- Garlic scapes
- Ginger
- Gooseberries
- Gourd
- Grape tomato
- Green Beans
- Habanero chili
- Heart of palm
- Horseradish
- Jalapeño
- Jerusalem artichoke/Sunchoke
- Jicama
- Kale
- Leeks
- Lemon
- Lentils

- Lemongrass
- Lettuce
- Lime
- Lotus root
- Marjoram
- Melons
- Mushrooms
- Mustard Greens
- Napa cabbage
- Okra
- Onions
- Olives
- Parsley
- Parsnips
- Peas
- Plantain
- Poblano pepper
- Pumpkins
- Quince
- Radicchio
- Radish
- Rainbow chard
- Red cabbage
- Rhubarb
- Romaine lettuce
- Romanesco
- Rosemary
- Rutabaga
- Savoy cabbage
- Scallions/Spring onions
- Seaweed
- Shallots
- Snow peas
- Sorrel
- Spaghetti squash
- Spinach
- Sprouts
- Squash
- Squash blossoms/flowers
- Sweet potato
- Sugar snap peas
- Taro
- Thyme
- Tomatillo
- Tomato
- Turnips
- Vidalia onions
- Wasabi
- Water chestnut
- Watercress
- Watermelon
- White eggplant
- White onion
- Yellow squash
- Zucchini/Courgette

FRUITS

- Acai
- Apple
- Apricot
- Avocado
- Banana
- Bilberry
- Bitter gourd
- Blackberry
- Blackcurrant
- Blood Orange
- Blueberry
- Cantaloupe
- Carob
- Chayote
- Cherry
- Chestnut
- Clementines
- Cloudberry
- Cranberry
- Cucumber
- Dragonfruit
- Durian
- Elderberry
- Gooseberry
- Grapefruit
- Grapes
- Guava
- Honeydew
- Huckleberry
- Jackfruit
- Jujube
- Juniper berry
- Kaffir lime
- Kiwi
- Kumquat
- Lemons
- Lingonberry
- Loganberry
- Lucuma
- Lychee
- Mandarin
- Mangosteen
- Monk Fruit
- Mulberry
- Nectarines
- Nutmeg
- Orangelo
- Orange
- Papaya
- Passion Fruit
- Peach
- Pear
- Persimmon
- Plum/Plumcot
- Pluot
- Pomegranate
- Pummelo
- Rambutan
- Raspberry
- Star Fruit
- Tamarind
- Tangerine
- Tomato
- Ugli
- Watermelon

BEANS, LEGUMES & NUTS

- Alfalfa
- Anasazi beans
- Azuki beans
- Bean sprouts
- Black beans
- Black-eyed peas
- Broad beans
- Cannellini beans
- Fava beans
- Garbanzo beans
- Green beans
- Kidney beans
- Lentils
- Lima beans
- Mung beans
- Navy beans
- Northern beans
- Peas
- Pinto beans
- Red beans
- Tamarind beans
- Wax beans

- White beans
- Almond
- Almond butter
- Beech
- Brazil Nuts
- Breadnut
- Candlenut
- Cashews
- Chestnuts
- Chia seed
- Flaxseed
- Hazelnut
- Hickory nuts
- Kola nut
- Macadamia
- Pecans
- Pine nut
- Pistachio
- Poppyseed
- Pumpkin seed
- Sunflower seed
- Walnut

ANIMAL PRODUCTS

- Bass
- Beef
- Chicken
- Clams
- Cod
- Crab
- Duck
- Eggs
- Flounder
- Halibut
- Ham
- Lamb
- Lobster
- Mussels
- Octopus
- Oyster
- Pork
- Ribs
- Salmon
- Sardines
- Scallop
- Sea bass
- Shrimp
- Sole
- Steak
- Swordfish
- Trout
- Tuna
- Turkey

MEAL PLAN

Here is a meal plan you can use as inspiration for your new diet based on the above lists. Remember that the food elimination list applies, so you should not add sugar, dairy, or wheat ingredients to any of the meals below. A good idea is to choose a meal that you are interested in cooking from the plan below, then search for recipes that are gluten free and dairy free.

This meal plan was designed to show you that you can have delicious, exciting food without sugar and bread. I hope it helps you!

DAY 1:
Breakfast: Spinach Frittata with Warm Spiced Almond Milk (Ground Turmeric, Ginger, and Cinnamon)
Lunch: Green Salad with Sliced Boiled Eggs, Bell Peppers, and Onion dressed with Tuna, Avocado, Olive Oil and Vinegar
Dinner: Herb and Walnut-Crusted Fish with Grilled Vegetables

DAY 2:
Breakfast: Warm Applesauce with Cinnamon
Lunch: Shrimp and Broccoli Stir-Fry, Ginger, and Scallions
Dinner: Cauliflower Rice with Kale, Roasted Garlic, and Black Beans

DAY 3:
Breakfast: Two Hard-Boiled Eggs, Almond Butter Squeeze Pack
Lunch: Chipotle Pepper Marinated Grilled Chicken and Smoky Chickpea Salad (Chickpeas, Sweet Bell Peppers, Lemon Juice, Olive Oil, Smoked Paprika)
Dinner: Roasted Lemon Dill Salmon and Steamed Seasonal Vegetables

DAY 4:
Breakfast: Sunnyside Up Eggs with Salsa Verde and Black Beans
Lunch: Grilled Steak over Arugula and Cherry Tomatoes with Balsamic Vinaigrette
Dinner: Zucchini Noodles with Homemade Tomato Sauce and Black Pepper

DAY 5:
Breakfast: Warm Flax Pudding made with Almond Milk, topped with Cooked Berry Compote
Lunch: Turkey Meatball Lettuce Wrap with Smashed Sweet Potatoes
Dinner: Stuffed Bell Pepper filled with Quinoa and Vegetables

DAY 6:
Breakfast: Poached Eggs with Roasted Crispy Kale and Pumpkin Seeds
Lunch: Grilled Salmon with Grilled Asparagus
Dinner: Chopped Salad with Baked Falafel, Tomato, Radishes, and Cucumber with Hummus

DAY 7:
Breakfast: Chia Seed Pudding with Sliced Bananas and Melted Almond Butter
Lunch: Roasted Vegetable Buddha Bowl (Brussel Sprouts, Peppers, Carrots, Kale) with Dairy-Free Creamy Cashew Dressing
Dinner: Chicken Meatballs with Garlic and Black Pepper Spaghetti Squash

DAY 8:
Breakfast: Two Eggs Sunny Side Up with Salmon and Half a Grapefruit
Lunch: Spinach Soup with Cauliflower, Cabbage, and Onions
Dinner: Mung Bean and Quinoa Kitchari with Broccoli and Carrots

DAY 9:
Breakfast: Hummus with Carrot and Celery Sticks, and Sunflower Seed Butter Almond Milk Smoothie
Lunch: Shrimp and Veggie Lettuce Wraps (carrots, peppers, bean sprouts)
Dinner: Vegetarian Three-Bean Chili

DAY 10:
Breakfast: Broccoli and Tomato Frittata
Lunch: Turkey, Sprout, and Hummus Collard Wrap with Julienned Vegetables
Dinner: Beet and Squash Gnocchi with Sautéed Rainbow Chard

DAY 11:
Breakfast: Spiced Chicken Scramble with Black Beans
Lunch: Spinach Salad topped with Grilled Shrimp

Dinner: Chimichurri Marinated Chicken Kebabs with Slow-Roasted Tomatoes

DAY 12:
Breakfast: Eggs and Turkey Bacon, Banana Smoothie
Lunch: Chicken Meatballs over Chive Cauliflower Mash
Dinner: Zucchini Noodles with Beet Walnut Pesto and Roasted Carrots

DAY 13:
Breakfast: Mushroom and Caramelized Onion Omelette
(Onions Caramelized with Grapeseed or Avocado Oil, No Sugar)
Lunch: Lemon, Shallot, and Herb Quinoa
Dinner: Onion, Celery, and Bell Pepper Stuffed Baked Clams with Almond Milk Creamed Spinach

DAY 14:
Breakfast: Green Smoothie (spinach, banana, flax seeds, coconut milk)
Lunch: Steak Salad with Chickpeas and Avocado Cilantro Dressing
Dinner: Escarole and Beans

DAY 15:
Breakfast: Sardines with Mango
Lunch: Lentil Soup
Dinner: Salmon Cakes with Dijon Drizzle, Capers, and Toasted Almond Asparagus

DAY 16:
Breakfast: Poached Eggs over Cauliflower Hash Browns with Bacon and Leeks
Lunch: Grilled Chicken with White Bean Salad
Dinner: Hearty Vegetable Borscht

DAY 17:
Breakfast: Chia Pudding with Mango Puree and Warm Ginger Tea
Lunch: Chicken Thighs over Quinoa with Collard Greens
Dinner: Shredded Barbecue Codfish with Cabbage Slaw

DAY 18:
Breakfast: Avocado Egg Cup with Fresh Tomato Salsa
Lunch: Cauliflower Tortilla Wrap with White Beans and Roasted Peppers
Dinner: Lemon Oil Grilled Steak with Seasonal Vegetable Ratatouille

DAY 19:
Breakfast: Two Hard-Boiled Eggs with Sausage and Almond Butter Banana Smoothie
Lunch: Dairy-Free Baba Ganoush with Vegetables
Dinner: Sesame Shrimp and Broccoli Bowl with Mushrooms

DAY 20:
Breakfast: Sunny Side Up Egg and Avocado Mash on Cauliflower Toast, with Rosewater and Cardamom Spiced Almond Milk
Lunch: Quinoa Buddha Bowl with Swiss Chard, Carrots, Broccoli, and Charred Scallions
Dinner: Taco Bowl with Chipotle Chicken, Fajita Vegetables, Lettuce, Tomatoes, Guacamole, and Cilantro

DAY 21:
Breakfast: Overnight Flax Chia Pudding with Blackberry Sauce and Coconut Flakes
Lunch: Steak with Mushroom Gravy and Cauliflower Mash
Dinner: Spinach Salad with Edamame, Microgreens, and Cucumber with Avocado Green Goddess Dressing

DAY 22:
Breakfast: Tomato and Basil Frittata with Sautéed Asparagus
Lunch: Turkey Meatloaf with Roasted Brussels Sprouts
Dinner: Winter Vegetable Bake with Acorn Squash, Carrots, Sweet Potatoes, Beets, and Garlic

DAY 23:
Breakfast: Vegan Mango Lassi (Mango, Light Coconut Milk, Soaked Cashews Blended) and Raw Mixed Nuts
Lunch: Pan-Roasted Chicken Thighs with String Bean, Chickpea, and Tomato Salad
Dinner: French Lentil Vegetable Soup

DAY 24:
Breakfast: 2-Ingredient Pancakes (Bananas and Eggs) with Bacon
Lunch: Pan-Seared Scallops with Lemon Caper Pan Sauce and Parsnip Rutabaga Mash
Dinner: Sautéed Kale and White Bean Salad with Walnuts and Lemon Tahini (Sesame Seeds Blended with Grapeseed Oil)

DAY 25:
Breakfast: Chicken Sausage and Cabbage with Warm Apple Sauce
Lunch: Baked Salmon with Avocado Salsa and Arugula Salad
Dinner: Artichoke Heart and Caramelized Onion Frittata

DAY 26:
Breakfast: Avocado Mash on Cauliflower Toast and Turmeric Spiced Almond Milk
Lunch: Chicken Breast Stuffed with Spinach with Herbed Quinoa
Dinner: Almond Flour and Flax Crusted Fish with Baked String Beans and Cauliflower

DAY 27:
Breakfast: Shakshuka
Lunch: Garlic Shrimp and Bok Choy Stir-Fry with Ginger and Peppers
Dinner: Ribs with Mashed Sweet Potatoes and Romaine and Cucumber Salad

DAY 28:
Breakfast: Almond Butter and Fruit Smoothie (strawberry, blueberry, almond butter, banana)
Lunch: Turkey Burger with Sweet Potato "Bun" and Crispy Kale Chips
Dinner: Smoky Black Beans with Baked Plantains

DAY 29:
Breakfast: Blended Berry Bowl with Grainless Granola, Almond Butter, Pineapple, and Mango
Lunch: Grilled Chicken with Fennel, Radicchio, and Clementine Salad
Dinner: Jackfruit Stuffed Portobello Mushrooms with Kale Cabbage Slaw

DAY 30:
Breakfast: Cauliflower Tortilla Breakfast Burrito with Scrambled Eggs, Quinoa, Beans, Vegetables, and Salsa
Lunch: French Onion Soup
Dinner: Crockpot Pulled Barbecue Chicken in a Lettuce Wrap

DAY 31:
Breakfast: Banana Raspberry Breakfast Bars
Lunch: Salmon Meatballs with Dijon Lemon Sauce and Chopped Chives
Dinner: Cauliflower Steak with Black Quinoa and Roasted Beets

DAY 32:
Breakfast: Grilled Chicken with apples and carrots
Lunch: Baked Fish with broccoli and cauliflower
Dinner: Salad with Romaine, onions, peppers, carrots, cucumbers, tomatoes, and celery

DAY 33:
Breakfast: Baked Fish with Onions, Peppers, Tomatoes, and Mango
Lunch: Turkey Balls with Asparagus
Dinner: Eggplant with tomatoes and squash

DAY 34:
Breakfast: Salmon with a side of Sliced Bananas and Grapes
Lunch: Organic Burger with Sliced Red Peppers as the buns with lettuce tomatoes onions and pickles
Dinner: Cabbage Soup with onions, broccoli, celery, squash, zucchini, peppers, onion, garlic,

DAY 35:
Breakfast: Eggs with Kale, Mushrooms, and Cucumbers
Lunch: Quinoa with black beans and carrots peas
Dinner: Lettuce Wraps with Sliced chicken and veggies

SNACK IDEAS
1. Portioned Leftovers
2. Sliced Apples and Bananas with Almond Butter
3. Mixed Fruit/Fruit Salad
4. 2-3 Dates
5. Raw Almonds, Cashews, or Brazil Nuts
6. Raw Carrots, Cauliflower, and Celery with Hummus
7. Vegetables with Guacamole
8. Avocado on a Cauliflower Tortilla
9. Baked Apple Chips
10. Banana "Ice Cream" (frozen bananas and almond milk in food processor)
11. Celery Sticks with Almond Butter
12. Oven-baked Zucchini Chips
13. Oven-baked Kale Chips
14. Green Beans

15. Hard-boiled Eggs
16. Egg Cups
17. Pomegranate
18. Snap Peas
19. Turkey Roll-ups
20. Grapes
21. Toasted Pumpkin Seeds
22. Oven-toasted Chickpeas
23. Grainless Granola—chopped pecans, almonds, sunflower seeds, and dried apples
24. Carrots
25. Nut Bars
26. Fruit Bars
27. Veggie Sticks

Recipes

When first adapting to a new diet, it is sometimes difficult to figure out what kinds of foods to eat. Here are some simple and delicious recipes that can help you transition into a new way of eating. We are sure you'll find that these recipes are just as tasty as the foods you used to enjoy; only they have the added benefit of making you feel great!

BREAKFAST:

Banana and Almond Butter Overnight Chia Pudding
- 1 ½ cups non-dairy unsweetened plant milk
- 3 tablespoons high-quality chia seeds
- 1 vanilla bean pod
- 2 ripe banana
- ⅛ cup almonds
- ½ cup organic, unsweetened almond butter

The night before, mix the plant milk and chia seeds together. Scrape out the seeds from the vanilla pod and mix these in. Let this sit in the refrigerator for 12 hours or overnight.

In the morning, heat the almond butter in a pan until it melts slightly. Add 1 cup of chia pudding to a bowl and pour the almond butter over it. Slice the banana and put it on top. Sprinkle the almonds on top and enjoy!

Huevos Rancheros with Salsa Verde and Refried Beans

- 2 eggs
- Olive, coconut, avocado, or grapeseed oil

Salsa Verde:

- 3 pounds fresh tomatillos (green tomatoes)
- 6-9 serrano chilies
- 2-3 cloves garlic
- ¼ cup olive, grapeseed, or avocado oil
- 1 tbsp. pink sea salt

Refried Beans:

- 1-2 tbsp olive, grapeseed, or avocado oil
- ½ yellow onion
- 1 tsp chili powder
- ¼ tsp cayenne pepper
- 1 ½ cups cooked pinto beans
- ½ cup chicken stock or vegetable stock
- salt and pepper to taste

- 2-3 sprigs cilantro

Make the salsa verde first by boiling tomatillos and serrano chilies in water for approximately 15 minutes or until tender and dull in color. Drain and transfer to a blender. Add garlic and blend into a smooth sauce. Heat the oil in a pan, then pour in the sauce and cook, stirring constantly until it bubbles. Simmer until the consistency is slightly thicker. Add salt to taste.

To make the beans, add oil to a pan, then dice and sauté the onions until cooked through. Then add chili powder and cayenne pepper. Add the cooked beans and stock, then mash with a potato masher or back of a spoon. Add salt and pepper to taste.

TO ASSEMBLE:

Cook the eggs to your liking and plate them over the salsa verde with the refried beans on the side. Top with cilantro, and feel free to garnish with pico de gallo.

Fresh Cinnamon Applesauce

Cook diced apples in just enough water to cover them and add cinnamon and ground ginger to taste. Immediately blend this in a bullet blender and enjoy fresh, warm cinnamon applesauce!

LUNCH OR DINNER:

The Best Simple Green Salad

- 2 hard-boiled eggs, sliced
- Spinach, spring mix, green leaf lettuce, etc.
- 1-2 bell peppers, sliced into strips
- 1 red onion, sliced
- 1 avocado, cut into chunks
- 1 portion high-quality tuna
- Olive oil and red wine vinegar to dress salad
- Salt and pepper to taste

Add lettuce and greens to a large bowl. Slice eggs, peppers, onions, and avocado and add to bowl. Add tuna, and then drizzle with vinegar and oil and dress. The tuna and avocado should mix with the oil and vinegar to create a dressing. Finally, freshly grind some black pepper over the salad and add pink sea salt to taste.

Vegetarian Bean Chili

- Olive oil, grapeseed oil, or avocado oil
- 1 medium onion
- 1 large bell pepper
- 3 large carrots, chopped
- 3 ribs celery, chopped
- ½ teaspoon salt
- 3 cloves garlic
- 2 tbsp chili powder
- 2 tsp cumin
- 2 tsp smoked paprika
- 1 tsp dried oregano

- 28 ounces diced tomatoes with juices
- 30 ounces black beans
- 15 ounces pinto beans
- 2 cups vegetable broth
- 1-2 teaspoons vinegar

Garnish:

- Cilantro
- Avocado
- Raw tomatoes

Heat the oil then add onion, pepper, carrots, celery, and salt. Cook until everything is cooked and tender. Next, add the garlic, spices, and oregano.

Add the tomatoes, beans, and broth. Bring to a boil, then lower the heat and simmer gently for 30 minutes. Mash this until it thickens to the desired texture. Mix in the vinegar. Garnish as desired and enjoy!

Herb and Walnut-Crusted Fish

- ½ pound of good quality wild fish (cod, halibut)
- ⅓ cup walnuts, finely chopped
- ¼ cup fresh parsley
- 2-3 sprigs of fresh thyme
- Olive oil as needed
- 2 tbsp lemon juice
- 1 tbsp lemon zest

Preheat the oven to 425 degrees. Lightly coat a pan with olive oil and place the fish fillets on the pan. Drizzle with lemon juice.

Next, make the crust. Place the walnuts, thyme, a splash of olive oil, lemon zest, and a squeeze or two of lemon juice in a food processor or bullet blender. Pulse until a coarse mixture forms. Press this mixture onto the top of each piece of fish. Then bake for approximately 15 minutes or until the fish is flaky.

Serve with quinoa salad or grilled vegetables.

DESSERT:

Date and Fresh Cut Fruit Salad

- Pitted dates
- Seasonal fruits, cut
  examples:
  pineapple
  cantaloupe
  watermelon
  apples
  orange slices
  cherries
  berries

Slice all the fruits and add to a bowl with the pitted dates. Share with a friend!

These are just some ideas. There are so many great books and resources of recipes and healthy eating ideas. Keep in mind; you do not have to be creative. Quick and easy meals include baked fish, grilled chicken, turkey balls, scrambled eggs, steamed broccoli and cauliflower, raw salad, fruit platters, and homemade trail mixes. Quick and easy snacks include celery with almond butter, carrots with hummus, apple slices, strawberries and blueberries, oranges with pumpkin seeds, and grapes with walnuts.

Chapter 3: Chemical Imbalance

Another cause of brain dysfunction that can eventually lead to memory problems is chemical exposure. Chemicals are everywhere we go and are in almost every product we use. We live in a world of long ingredient lists, highly engineered products, and deceptive marketing. Many years ago, fruits and vegetables could be trusted. Harsh pesticides had not yet been developed and plants had not been scientifically genetically modified. Now, even simple foods like eggs bear the effects of being produced by chickens fed antibiotics and inappropriate diets. Companies that make the products we use typically do not have our health in mind, so we need to do our own research to make sure that the products we're using on our bodies and in our homes are not sabotaging our efforts for better health.

Most conventional cleaning products are filled with harsh and dangerous ingredients that can be replaced with equally efficient and cost-effective alternatives made from harmless household products like vinegar, baking soda, water, lemon, and essential oils. A quick search on the internet yields hundreds of recipes for homemade cleaners for laundry, kitchen surfaces, and bathrooms. You can personalize your cleaning supplies with essential oils you enjoy, like tea tree oil or lavender. If you like using air fresheners at home, try essential oil diffusers instead—they are a great alternative to chemical-loaded air freshener sprays.

It is also crucial to be mindful of potentially toxic chemicals in our food to which many people expose themselves several times each day. The vast majority of conventional produce in grocery stores has been genetically modified or exposed to powerful pesticides. Seeking out organic options or buying produce from farmers' markets can reduce your exposure to these toxic chemicals.

At home, make sure you're cooking your organic produce on coating-free cookware. Cast iron and stainless steel are much safer than non-stick pots and pans and work just as well. Chemicals are also found in many kinds of food-storage containers. In plastic containers, even if the product says BPA-free, there are still other chemicals that can be absorbed into your food. I recommend storing all your food in glass containers. It is heavier but much healthier.

We must also be aware of the chemicals in our drinking water. Tap water can contain chlorine, fluoride or lead that can be harmful to your health. If possible, you should invest in a high-quality water filter, since most popular water filters have limitations on what chemicals they are able to filter. Bottled water is not the solution because most water comes in plastic bottles that leak chemicals into the water. Leaving water bottles outside in the sun or in the car makes this problem even worse. Reusing old water bottles increases the quantity of chemical seepage. The best solution is to get a water filter at home that attaches under the sink as well as to the showerhead. I recommend a high-quality, heavy-duty filter that removes lead, aluminum, and fluoride. After it's installed, invest in some glass bottles and use these to store and transport your drinking water. This way, you can avoid the plastic in the bottles as well as heavy metals from the tap.

Antiperspirant is another common way people expose themselves to heavy metals every day. The danger of antiperspirant is primarily aluminum, which attacks your nervous system and has been tied to degenerative brain disease. Aluminum is one of the leading causes of Alzheimer's disease and can even lead to breast cancer, as well. To protect your memory as you age, it is absolutely necessary that you cut aluminum-containing products out of your life. Antiperspirant is very bad for your body. It clogs up the sweat glands, preventing our bodies from detoxing. Sweating is a healthy, natural bodily process. If we don't sweat, then we cannot get rid of the harsh toxins in our body. We need to detox! Humans detox by means of sweat, vomit, urination, defecation, mucus production, tears, and menstruation, to name a few examples. Drinking clean water is one of the best ways to detox naturally. My patients always say, "But if I drink more water, then I'll need to pee more," and my response is always, "Yes, that's right!" More frequent urination is a good thing because peeing is crucial to get rid of waste in the body.

Cosmetics are another major culprit of repeated chemical exposure. Lotion, body wash, shampoo, and makeup can all be harmful to your health. Some beauty products contain formaldehyde, which has been shown to have negative effects on the nervous system, lungs, nose, and throat, and may potentially also cause cancer. Ironically, sunscreen is one of the most toxic cosmetic products available, but that does not mean you should stop using sunscreen! Visit our website *www.kaplandc.com* for recommendations on healthy sunscreen and beauty-supply options. If you use a product on your body, it is worthwhile to do some research to find out if it contains ingredients that could harm you.

Many products that have been developed more recently in history are full of chemically engineered ingredients. There is no perfect way of knowing if these products are safe for long-term use. The best way to start is to take a step back and think about the products you use. How many cosmetics do I have? How many cleaning supplies do I have? How many ingredients on this bottle have I never heard of? Do I really need to put this product on my body, inside my home, or in my breathing air? If so, are there any good alternatives that are safer or cleaner? If you ask yourself these questions and start avoiding harsh chemicals, your brain will start functioning better, and you'll start feeling and living better. Remember that most of these chemicals can be replaced with cheaper and safer products like baking soda, lemon, and vinegar.

Chapter 4: Sleep Like a Log

We should be sleeping approximately one-third of our life. Since there are twenty-four hours in a day, that means we should be sleeping approximately eight hours a night. In addition, the most important hours of sleep are the hours before midnight. A good night's sleep will be from 10 p.m. to 6 a.m. in the winter and 10 p.m. to 5 a.m. in the summer. It is important to get a little more sleep in the winter as our body goes into a "mini-hibernation."

Many of my patients tell me that they stay up late watching TV, Netflix, movies, YouTube, or the news. If they are not in front of the big flat-screen TV, they are scrolling through Instagram and Facebook or playing on the computer when they could be in bed sleeping. Going to bed late will lead to anxiety and an increase in stress levels, which can be one of the contributing factors in memory loss. Furthermore, watching television, you may find yourself exposed to junk food advertising that could cause you to start snacking late at night. One of the easiest ways to lose weight is to get to bed at least two hours before midnight and turn off the TV, especially the news. This will decrease your belly fat by reducing cortisol levels.

If you want to get to bed earlier, it is also important to avoid eating late at night. The most effective way to accomplish this is through intermittent fasting. Intermittent fasting can be defined as eating for eight hours (between the times of 9 a.m. and 5 p.m.) and fasting for sixteen hours (from 5 p.m. to 9 a.m.) The fasting period gives your body ample time to process the food you have already eaten and helps improve your quality of sleep. The purpose of eating is to accumulate energy. Given this information, eating late at night doesn't make sense! Why give yourself more energy at nighttime? It will only make falling asleep and staying asleep more difficult.

It is good to be in bed, but even more important is to get good, quality sleep. One way to improve the quality of your sleep is exercise. A good exercise routine will tire out your body and help you sleep better at night. And remember, the best time to exercise is in the morning, while cortisol levels are highest. Changing your lifestyle to get to bed earlier will have you naturally waking up earlier, and you can use those early morning hours to get some great exercise.

Another important factor in getting quality sleep is reducing blue light exposure. Blue light can be found on your computer, cell phone, TV, iPad, and other electronic devices. It is recommended you cease all electronic use after 5 p.m. Once you clock out of work, put the electronics away. They expose you to harmful blue light that stimulates cortisol, the stress hormone that disrupts proper sleep patterns and circadian rhythms. Cortisol also destroys cells in the hippocampus, which will lead to memory loss. If you have a job that requires a lot of staring at screens, invest in blue-light-blocking glasses. While you sleep, keep your Wi-Fi and cell phone off and your cell phone out of your room.

The key is to get into a really deep sleep, which is called the rapid eye movement (REM) phase. We should not have to wake up in the middle of the night to pee or rollover or check the time on our cell phones. We should wake up in the morning saying, "How long have I been out?" or even, "What day is it?" That is a deep sleep. We should also be able to wake up on our own and not to an alarm clock. Following the recommendations above will help you get a good night's sleep with plenty of REM, which will rejuvenate and re-oxygenate your brain to keep it healthy, boost your brainpower, and improve memory and focus.

Chapter 5: Keep Your Head Above Water

I had a patient, who we'll call Maria for privacy purposes, who came into the office with her daughter to improve her memory and focus. Her memory had declined so much that she could not answer simple questions like, "What is your age?" "What is the day of the week?" or "Can you name a fruit?" We urgently needed to figure out how to help her.

Based on her blood work and her history of avoiding drinking water, I knew that we needed to get her to start hydrating to help boost her brain. However, she refused to drink water, so we needed to get creative. Collaborating with her daughter, we figured out that if we took some water and mixed it with a fruit smoothie, she enjoyed hydrating much more. We began making smoothies with mangoes, strawberries, and other fruits (with all the fiber) and mixed in water so that they were about one-third fruit and two-thirds water.

Through this method, we quickly got Maria drinking the proper amount of water for her bodyweight, and within just a few days, the changes in her memory were dramatic. There was an amazing fifty-percent improvement in her brain function when performing certain brain tests such as a VNG and CAPS. By the end of the week, she was able to name about seven different fruits. She was able to tell me what state she was in and who was president— questions that only resulted in a blank face before increasing her water intake. She even remembered her daughter's name, causing her daughter to cry. Her life and the lives of her family improved so much just by drinking more water. That is the power of hydration for the brain.

The Earth is made up of 71 percent water. Our bodies are made up of 78 percent water when we are born and usually about 60 percent as we get older. Water is life. To stay hydrated, drink the same number of ounces as the number of your bodyweight halved, every day. For example, if you weigh 200 pounds, you should be drinking 100 ounces of water every day. I recommend drinking water with pink Himalayan salt, which contains 86 minerals. That is about half of all the minerals we have found on Earth. To balance out your electrolytes, I recommend getting a big salt rock and pouring your water over the rock into a container to help avoid putting too much salt in your water.

Water is the best source of hydration for our bodies. There are many beverages in the store that claim to provide "better hydration," but often these are packed with sugar, artificial flavors, food dyes, and other harmful chemicals—not to mention that they are typically packed in plastic bottles, which are bad for you and the environment. Avoid electrolyte drinks (Pedialyte or Gatorade), and certainly avoid soda and coffee. None of these drinks count as water. In fact, coffee dehydrates you, so if you do drink coffee, you must add an extra glass of water to the amount you drink that day.

People are usually surprised when I tell them to stop drinking fruit juices. Fruit juices contain all of the sugar and none of the fiber of the fruit. Smoothies are a better option if you enjoy having fruit in the morning, but do not remove any of the pulp.

You should also find out about the water quality in your home and community. Does it have a lot of fluoride, lead, or chlorine? If so, you should invest in a high-quality water filter designed to filter out these harmful chemicals. Typical water filters won't cut it. This does not just go for your drinking water; you can also be exposed to chemicals in the water when you shower or bathe. Many companies can install water filters for your shower as well. You should take an active interest to find out what is in your water in the first place, how dangerous some of these additives, chemicals, and heavy metals may be, and which steps you need to take to protect yourself from them.

As far as hydration, *when* you drink water is almost as important as simply ensuring you drink it. We should be drinking two glasses of warm lemon water when we wake up, as well as a glass thirty minutes before breakfast, thirty minutes before lunch, thirty minutes before dinner, and right before bed. Don't drink water after a meal because it dilutes the food, making it harder to digest. Instead, drinking water before meals has been shown to help lubricate the alimentary tract, making digestion more efficient and thereby helping people lose weight. After a workout, remember to replenish your fluids by drinking water. If you are on your period, drinking more water will help prevent PMS, cramping, and irritability. If you drink alcohol, I recommend having a glass of water for each drink you consume to keep your brain and body hydrated. This will not only be helpful for your brain and body in the long run, but will also help prevent a hangover the next day.

Many headaches are due to dehydration. If you frequently suffer from headaches, consider your water intake. Odds are, you are not drinking enough water. So don't take an aspirin; instead, enact a plan and set goals to drink more water. For instance, try to drink half of your daily water goal by noon. Use a big glass water bottle and keep it within reach.

Keeping the brain hydrated helps to maximize and unleash the brain's potential. Keep it hydrated, and your brain will function at optimal levels. Think of the brain as a grape. If you do not give it enough water, it will shrink and shrivel up and turn into a raisin. Do not let this happen to your brain. The key to any disease is prevention. Keep your brain and body strong with this simple, easy, and affordable solution. And keep in mind, water also makes your hair and skin look beautiful and helps improve libido, digestion, circulation, energy, and sleep.

Chapter 6: Love Conquers All

The human need for community and interaction is not just sentimental. The brain truly needs this type of stimulation to boost your brainpower. This need for community was researched in prisons, and they discovered that people who are in solitary confinement start to experience a quick decline in health. These prisoners hate being alone so much that they actually prefer to be next to murderers and violent criminals rather than in solitary. Because the brain needs interaction, communication, and social activity, prisoners will do anything to avoid this punishment.

In regard to brain function, it doesn't matter how many Facebook friends you have, but rather how many in-person social experiences you have with friends or family. People are fooled into thinking they are being social because they are getting "likes" and comments on social media. We should actually call it "anti-social media" because it is preventing us from having face-to-face interactions. If patients tell me that they have no friends or family, then I let them know it is important to make some friends. If you really think it is too hard and there is absolutely no way you could ever make a new friend, you might choose to have a meaningful relationship with a pet. If you can't get a pet, try a doll. In *Castaway*, for instance, Tom Hanks's character personified a volleyball to talk to and interact with, and that relationship saved his brain.

My suggestion is to get off your phone, stop sitting at home on the computer or watching TV, and go out into the real world. If you don't have a friend to go out with, just walk outside and enjoy some people watching. You might see people sitting at a cafe having their first date, an old married couple holding hands walking down the street, kids hanging out together, or a mother strolling with her baby. Watching these activities activates mirror neurons that will stimulate the brain as much as doing the activities yourself.

Another idea is to stop wishing people a happy birthday on

Facebook, and instead pick up the phone. They will appreciate it so much more. You can hear a smile over the phone, and that will stimulate your brain. Don't send a text telling someone you love them; send them a card. They will probably never read that text again, but they will keep the card. Don't buy people presents for their birthdays; do something special like taking a painting class together, going to a Broadway show, or going to Rockefeller Center to ice skate! Make a memory together rather than buying some materialistic gift. And keep all your memories in a book. That way, if you are having a bad day or are feeling anxious or depressed, you can flip through the book, and it will light up your day, releasing endorphins that will give you a natural high to get you out of that funk. Life is a collection of memories, not a collection of things.

It might be hard to believe, but staying connected is an extremely important step to boosting brainpower. Staying engaged with people and having good, positive, face-to-face interactions, or getting out into the world and spending time in your community stimulates the brain while maintaining its health and strength. Start spending more time with your family. Neuroscience has proven that grandparents who spend time with grandkids live longer and report an increase in overall happiness. This is the result of a symbiotic relationship. Grandparents share their experience, knowledge, and love with their grandkids, and in turn receive a brainpower boost— improving their happiness, health, and quality of life. But don't just think about it. In these modern times, you have to actually manage your calendar—not only for work, holidays, or special events, but for meeting up with friends and family. Social interaction is vital to boosting brain function.

Chapter 7: The More You Give,
the More You Receive

At the end of an appointment, I always ask my patients if they have any questions. One question I get occasionally, usually said in a joking manner, is, "What is the meaning of life?" I always respond the same way, "The meaning of life is to help other people and the planet." It's important to stop worrying or complaining about your life and to start helping people. Preliminary results from two Yale University studies have shown that people who harbor a lot of negativity, anger, and complaints are more likely to get Alzheimer's. If you start helping other people, you will boost your brainpower, thereby improving mood, memory, focus, and motivation. Go into every situation in life thinking of ways to help people. Maybe you can offer somebody a ride home, take out somebody's garbage, put someone's bag in the overhead compartment on an airplane, help someone move, drop someone off at the airport, or walk someone's dog for them. These are just a few ideas, but you get the gist.

I have noticed that people who complain the most tend to watch the news and use social media more frequently. Please don't waste your life watching TV and playing on the internet when you could instead be improving someone's day and improving your brain function. The news is designed to shock and upset people, drawing them in to watch more by emphasizing drama and fear. Social media is largely a collection of people sharing the positive or exciting parts of their lives. These posts can make you feel like your life has more conflict or negativity than your friends and family, but this is an illusion. Everyone faces some degree of trouble or suffering in their lives. Perform an experiment: stop watching the news and using social media for two weeks, and see how much better you feel.

Service is a great way to use your energy positively to help your community. Even if you have no money, you can make a change. When I was in college at Emory University, for instance, many people participated in a program called Habitat for Humanity, where college students help the less fortunate by building them houses. When I was in chiropractic school, many students would go to foreign countries on mission trips to give chiropractic adjustments to children and adults in need of care. These students adjusted hundreds of people a day and helped them with a variety of health problems. Volunteer initiatives are great ways to give back, help others, and build community. You can even get involved in organizing service trips at a local temple, church, or community center. Your time and talents can make a difference in someone's life.

If you are fortunate enough to have money to give to charity, remember that even a little can make a big difference in countries where resources are scarce. In many developing nations, people do not have ready access to clothes, shoes, or socks. Families in these countries cannot afford books, pencils, or paper, and sending their children to school is a huge financial hardship. Some hospitals in remote areas cannot afford scalpels, knives, and bandages. There are delivery services that provide large boxes with affordable shipping rates, thereby making it possible to buy many of these much-needed supplies at a dollar store and send them to little communities around the world for as little as a hundred dollars.

But remember, you do not need money to help people. If you know a lot about cars, help someone change a flat tire. If you are strong, help someone move heavy boxes. If someone is struggling with parking their car, offer your assistance. If someone is lost, give them directions. Or find something that you are passionate about and help people in your own way. Simply performing little acts of kindness every day can help. Whether it's opening the door for someone, picking up something that someone dropped, letting someone cut in front of you in line, walking an elderly woman across the street, or donating old clothes and shoes to the less fortunate, this action will create a "pay it forward" mentality that will help change your communities in positive ways. The less you complain and the more you give, the better your brain will function.

Chapter 8: Use It or Lose It

To boost your brainpower, we should focus on discovering any areas of the brain that have weak signals and addressing those specific areas to help them develop and function better. In my practice, we have technologically advanced equipment to diagnose areas of the brain that are not functioning at optimal levels. Using technologies like Videonystagmography (VNG), CAPS posturography, Interactive Metronome, electromyography, pulse oximetry, neurosensory integrators, and video balance boards, we can find areas of the brain that are not working properly and then come up with exercises that are proven through neuroscience to activate those specific areas of the nervous system.

For example, if the VNG finds that the frontal cortex is not firing properly, activating olfaction with smell while patients perform fine finger movements and fast eye movements can create neuroplastic changes through spatial and temporal summation. Spatial summation is when patients perform many exercises at the same time, and temporal summation is when they perform these exercises repeatedly to create long-term results. If the right frontal cortex is worse than the left frontal cortex in a hemispheric distribution, patients would only do the finger exercises on the left side, the quick eye movements to the left, and the smell only in the right nostril. The more specific you are with these neuroplasticity exercises, the better results you get. By utilizing proper brain exercises, we can help stop the beginning stages of frontotemporal dementia.

If an evaluation finds that the area of the brain called the parietal cortex is not working properly, it is most appropriate to do a type of therapy called proprioceptive exercises. For example, a doctor may draw letters on certain parts of the body while the patient, with his or her eyes closed, tries to correctly identify the letter. Another test has the doctor touch a specific point on the body, which patients must then touch while keeping their eyes closed. Or we might recommend balancing on one leg with your eyes closed, as this can only be done with good proprioception. A final example of a proprioceptive test is where we have patients identify different objects only by feeling with their hands or feet, while keeping their eyes closed. Brain exercises focused on identified weaknesses are very important to maximize your potential and maintain high functioning levels. We can provide this for all of the different areas of the brain.

If there are problems in a part of the brain called the temporal cortex, then memory tests, sound stimulation, and balance rehabilitation are recommended. If it is the occipital cortex that is not working well, then patients should focus on eye exercises. If the evaluation reveals problems with the fight-or-flight mode, neuroscience studies have proven that patients can stimulate their gag reflex or do gargling exercises to relax the nervous system by activating the vagus nerve. Certain facial massages, ear rubs, or even causing the eye to blink can activate the facial nerve, a part of the parasympathetic nervous system that helps you calm down, reduce your anxiety, and sleep better. Another way to activate the part of the brain that relaxes and rejuvenates is by performing specific eye exercises that research has shown may even help reduce high blood pressure and heart disease.

If the cerebellum is not functioning correctly, it is suggested that the patient perform coordination exercises by moving the arms and legs in complicated patterns like the infinity symbol, or we may rotate patients in a chair. If we aim to increase activation to the right cerebellum, we would spin them to the right or have them make complicated movements like drawing the infinity symbol using only the right arm. Therapies like these can improve balance, coordination, and help prevent falls. Although this is a lot of neuroscience talk, the main idea is that by doing neurological exercises focused on the weak areas of the nervous system, we can improve function in those areas and boost brainpower. You are only as strong as your weakest link, so although it is good to work on your strengths, it is equally as important to exercise the weaker parts of your brain.

My patients are always saying, "I exercise my brain because I do the crossword puzzle every day." Sure, that is a good start, but it may not be specific to the area of the brain that needs work. Because they do it every day, it probably isn't working on the weak areas, but only on areas that are already strong. That is why we do a proper evaluation to determine which specific area of the brain most needs work. People ask me about doing brain exercises on the computer, and I respond that brain exercises are best when they involve movement. The brain loves movement, so it is recommended you do activities where you are not sitting at a computer or using a tablet or phone rather than moving your body.

If you want to work your brain while sitting, make sure you change it up. Do the crossword puzzle on Monday, Word Jumble on Tuesday, Sudoku on Wednesday, Word Find on Thursday, Scrabble on Friday, Lumosity on Saturday, and Memory Match on Sunday. The brain loves new activities, and brain function increases with novelty.

Brain Exercises

Brain exercises are a great way for anyone to improve their memory and focus. Many of these exercises are relatively simple to do. It just takes dedication to develop the habit of doing the exercises three times a day.

TOP 7 BRAIN EXERCISES
TO IMPROVE MEMORY & FOCUS

1. CROSS CRAWL

- Think of a theme (colors, foods, animals, holiday's, presidents, etc.).
- Tap your left knee with their right hand and your right knee with your left hand - to every tap say an answer pertaining to the theme you selected
- Repeat this for 30 seconds

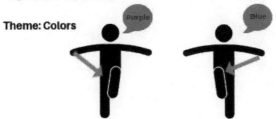

Theme: Colors

2. INFINITY SWING

- Draw the infinity symbol and trace over it without stopping or picking up your pen for 30 seconds

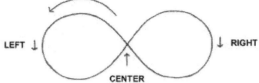

LEFT ↓   ↓ RIGHT

CENTER

3. SLAP, CHOP, FIST

- Using your non-dominant hand, repeat the sequence SLAP, CHOP, FIST for 30 seconds.
- When you get better at it, make the exercise harder by adding a scissor gesture.

4. GARGLING

- At least 3 times per day, gargle a sip of water for 30 seconds.
- Don't be dainty with this – gargle enthusiastically, make it challenging.
  This contracts the muscles in the back of the throat and activates the vagus nerve.

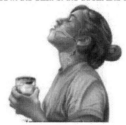

5. SMALL SACCADES

- Start with your eyes staring at the lower left dot. Count to three.
- On three, shift your eyes to the next dot going up the line.
- Repeat this for all the dots on the line.
- When finished, do the same thing starting from the lower right corner.

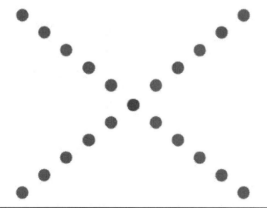

Chapter 9: Out with the Old, In with the New

As stated in the last chapter, do not be a creature of habit. Make sure you "switch it up." The brain does not like it if you are always doing the same thing. The top researchers and neuroscientists have found one of the top three ways to improve memory is to perform novel or new activities.

You must challenge your brain in different ways every single day. As mentioned, patients often tell me that they are challenging their brains because they do crossword puzzles or Sudoku every day. However, they are using the same parts of their brains and are strategizing the same way each time. Try a new game that you have never played before because as an alternate activity, it will require use of a different part of the brain.

Even the simple things in life should be done in a variety of ways. Patients are always telling me that they exercise, which, of course, is very good for the brain. However, many of them always exercise the same exact way. One patient told me she jogs five miles a day on the exact same path every single day. Although it is fantastic that she is running every day, it would be even better to jog one day, run one day, sprint one day, power walk one day, bike one day, swim one day, and rollerblade one day.

Another patient said he always runs on the treadmill on Monday, lifts weights for the upper body on Wednesday, and lifts weights for the lower body on Friday. Although I do commend him for working out three days a week, it is better to keep changing up the routine with weights, bands, or balls. I recommended he use the bike, the stair master, the elliptical, the rowing machine, the free weights, abdominal equipment, the pull-up bar, and other machines at his gym. Take different classes like Crossfit, Soul Cycle, Pilates, HIIT, Yoga, Tai Chi, Zumba, Hip-Hop Dance, Pole Dancing, Circuit Training, Boot Camp, P90X, and Insanity. There are so many ways to develop different muscles so that your brain is challenged in different ways.

Other novel activities that do not involve physical challenges include learning a different language, skill, or art form. If you only speak English, learn a new language. In my opinion, it would be best to start with Spanish. It has a similar alphabet and has some of the same word origins, which would make it very easy to learn. In addition to boosting your brainpower, learning Spanish is also extremely useful in modern-day America. However, if you really want to challenge your brain by learning a language that is very important in this world, it would be best to learn Mandarin, a Chinese language that utilizes an entirely new way of thinking. First of all, they do not use letters but symbols. Moreover, they traditionally read top to bottom rather than left to right. Another language you could learn that would switch things up and boost your brainpower is Hebrew. I recommend learning to read and write in Hebrew because understanding the Hebrew alphabet requires you to learn a completely new way of writing that English-speaking brains have never before experienced. Additionally, in Hebrew, you read from right to left rather than left to right, which uses more brainpower for those unaccustomed to the language. To really challenge your brain, try to read Hebrew without vowels, which requires even more focus and intention. Think of the brain as a muscle. You work your muscles hard to gain muscle mass. The same is true for the brain. You really have to work it hard to gain better brain function.

The point is to keep looking for novelty. There are so many novel activities that you can perform on a daily basis. You can start by taking a different route to work. Novelty can be applied to food, as well. Eat each color of the rainbow every day. Don't keep eating the same meals every day. Don't have a weekly menu. Change up the food you eat every day. Luckily, with the great variety of foods available to us, this task is very easy.

Find some new hobbies as well. For example, you can join a book club, take a salsa lesson, learn an instrument, take a sewing lesson, or participate in a cooking class. You might start gardening and learning about flowers. Go bird watching and study the different species of birds and all the different sounds they make. You can start a collection of stamps or baseball cards, where you are learning new facts. Start learning about cars, all their parts, how to fix them when they break, and how to maintain them. You could take up an interest in astronomy and research about the stars, planets, and galaxies.

Discover hobbies that you are passionate about and really enjoy. This way, you are having fun and learning at the same time.

In conclusion, it is important to change up every activity you do and to keep learning new things. Start brushing your teeth or your hair with your non-dominant hand. Walk sideways or backward occasionally. Meet new people and visit places you have never been to before. Perform activities you have never done. These simple changes will help you improve your memory, increase your brain function, improve your quality of life, and lead to a long healthy life with your family and friends.

Chapter 10: Everything Under the Sun

Many doctors will tell you to stay out of the sun. In my opinion, that is completely unwarranted unless you have a history of skin cancer. The key is not to overdo it, as we definitely need the sun to survive and thrive. We would all be dead without the sun. It assists us in boosting our brainpower and helps with growth, our bony structures, and thyroid function, just to name a few. If you are spending your vacation outside in the sun all day long, I suggest putting on specific brands of sunscreen to make sure you do not get burnt. However, most days, when you are inside and wearing clothes, there is no need for sun protection.

Suntan lotions and sunscreens are some of the most toxic products on the planet. Some commercial brands arc actually so strong they can erase permanent marker. What does that tell you about what it is doing to your skin? Thankfully, there are some companies developing sunblocks that are designed with fewer harsh chemicals to be safer for your body. Do not buy from chain stores like CVS, Walmart, or Target. Their products are full of toxins that cause brain and body inflammation, which is a "silent killer."

Another "silent killer" toxin can be found in our own atmosphere and is purposely created by the US Military. The government has a program called geo-engineering where chemicals are sprayed into the air to reflect sunlight away from the Earth in hopes of preventing global warming. However, there are two major problems with this. The first is that the chemicals they are spraying into the air invade our lungs, our water, our food, and our soil. The second problem is that we need the sun's rays.

One of the reasons the sun is so important is because of Vitamin D. Your blood work should show a vitamin D level above 50 ng/mL. Most labs will define over 30 ng/mL as normal; however, that "normal" is compared to people who work inside all day and never spend any time outside. That is not healthy. Every day we need to get vitamin D. Almost everyone gets a lunch break. Take this time to go outside, roll up your sleeves, take off your hat, get out of the shade, and stand in direct sunlight for twenty minutes a day with a lot of body exposure. Of course, throughout much of the year, it is too cold to do this properly, and it might be necessary to supplement. You may also want to supplement if you move somewhere like New Jersey or New York from a southern latitude like the Caribbean, South America, or Africa since your genetic makeup requires more Vitamin D to function at normal levels. Researchers have even proven that southern latitude offspring are more likely to develop neurological disorders like multiple sclerosis due to a vitamin D deficiency.

If you live somewhere in the northern latitudes, like New Jersey or New York, it is important to take Vitamin D supplements. The best product that I have researched is UltraD-5000 by Apex Energetics. In the winter, I personally take 10,000 IU a day, and in the summer, I take 5,000 IU a day. If your vitamin D levels are high, then your brain and thyroid functioning will improve, and you will be more likely to boost your brainpower. Conversely, if they are low, it may lead to brain, thyroid, and immune system dysfunction, as well as a major increase in depression.

Chapter 11: Take Two Aspirin and Call Me in the Morning

The average American takes twelve medications. In general, we are an over-medicated country. Medication takes a big toll on your health and will lead to suboptimal brain functioning. If you want to keep your brain healthy and prevent memory loss, it is important to take care of your body so that you do not have to take medication.

I understand that the United States has some of the best doctors in the world. If you have an emergency, you are in good hands in US hospitals. American doctors are the best at performing surgeries and prescribing medications. However, as students in medical school, they are not taught to be proficient in the prevention of disease. The four biggest health problems in America today are cancer, heart disease, Alzheimer's disease, and diabetes, and all four of these diseases can be *PREVENTED*. Don't wait until you get cancer and then have to receive chemotherapy. I have patients that have "chemo brain" and complain about memory loss. If you never get cancer in the first place, you will never need chemotherapy, and you won't suffer from "chemo brain." Do not wait until you get diabetes and have to take Metformin. Remember, diabetes is one of the leading causes of Alzheimer's disease. So, it is a good idea to cut out sugar, reduce carbohydrates, and start exercising to prevent your glucose levels from rising above the normal limit. Do not wait until you get heart disease and have to take blood pressure medication. Meditating daily, going to bed earlier, taking vacations, and avoiding sitting are key components in your heart health. Focusing on these strategies will help to keep your blood pressure in a healthy range, which is around 120/80 mm Hg. Stop eating dairy and bread products, so you do not get high cholesterol and then have to take Lipitor. These drugs have many side effects that affect the brain and will prevent you from maximizing your human potential.

Furthermore, some medications have side effects that require other medications. For example, I had a patient who we'll call John, who consumed a lot of bread, cheese, alcohol, and coffee, which caused acid reflux. He was prescribed an antacid to decrease the acid in his stomach. However, because his stomach acid decreased, he developed an overgrowth of bacteria in his stomach, which led to an infection. He then had to go on antibiotics. These antibiotics made him nauseous, so then he had to take a pill for his nausea. This is how taking one medication can lead to taking multiple medications. In my opinion, the best way of achieving optimal digestive health would be to avoid foods that cause acid reflux so that you never have to start taking medication in the first place.

So how can you prevent the four biggest diseases in America? Remember that cancer can be prevented by avoiding chemicals, focusing on stress reduction, and maintaining your immune system. Heart disease can be prevented by reducing inflammation, which in turn decreases the chances of a stroke or heart attack. Diabetes can be prevented with a great diet and exercise regime. If you prevent these three diseases, then you will avoid taking some extremely strong medications, and in turn, you will reduce your chances of developing brain issues like dementia or Alzheimer's.

Chapter 12: The Purpose of Life

You must have a purpose in your life—something you're working towards. My purpose is to improve people's health and well-being through functional neurology, functional medicine, chiropractic, physical therapy, herbal remedies, and educating the public on self-healing. Your purpose might be feeding the homeless, helping people with their health, writing books, designing buildings, teaching spirituality, painting, singing, making people laugh, or assisting people in making financial decisions. Your passion might be enlightening and motivating people, helping people exercise, or rescuing abandoned dogs. Everybody is different and has certain skills that will lead him or her down different pathways of life. Just remember that whatever path you take is the right one.

Maybe you have hobbies that make you happy and give your life meaning. Do you make art or music? Do you love crocheting or reading books? Everything from supporting a charity to learning carpentry or gardening can help keep your brain healthy. Perhaps you're passionate about caring for your friends or family. Maybe you advocate for a clean environment or spread the teachings of a religion.

Everyone can benefit from exploring a new interest. Consider taking an exercise class or joining a community group. Try going for a walk on a new trail or in another town. Take a music lesson or a cooking class. Do something new, spontaneous, and exciting! You never know what might wind up making your life bright. Your happiness and positive mood will be contagious, and before you know it, you will be spreading good energy wherever you go.

We all need a purpose, whether it helps other people or the planet. Your brain needs a reason to wake up in the morning and get moving. Your purpose should be something that you love to do and should require using your brain to plan, coordinate, organize, predict, remember, react, or take action. Doing things you love is an easy way to keep your brain working efficiently and effectively so that you can age happily.

Chapter 13: Sitting is the New Smoking

The Harvard study referenced in Chapter 1 suggested that sitting may have more influence on an early death than smoking. One of the reasons for this outcome is that people in the study who were smokers were not living a completely sedentary lifestyle. If their job required sitting, they made sure that they got up every twenty minutes. They might get a glass of water, go to the bathroom, get a fax, walk to the office down the hall, turn off the air conditioning, take a cigarette break, add paper to the copy machine, have a quick conversation with a coworker, or take a stretch break before going back to sitting. The point is that they did not sit all day. When comparing them to people who live a sedentary lifestyle, they actually live longer.

Sitting at work all day is bad for your brain and body, but remaining sedentary at home doubles the consequences. In addition to sitting at the computer every day from 9 a.m. to 5 p.m., some people sit on the subway, in a bus, or in their car during their commute. Afterward, they sit down and eat dinner. Then they sit on the couch and watch TV. Next, they sit down and spend time on their personal computers. Maybe they sit and read the newspaper or a good book. Finally, they might end the night by sitting and using their phones to browse social media or YouTube. When the weekend comes, they sit at the bar drinking, sit in the movie theatre, sit at the opera, sit during a dinner date, or sit at a Broadway play. Almost every activity people do involves sitting.

To keep your brain strong and healthy and to boost your brainpower, you must stay active. If you are in New York, take a walk along the High Line. Play tennis in Central Park. Go to the Bronx Zoo. Instead of taking the elevator, walk up the stairs. Instead of taking the subway, walk the twenty blocks. When you go to the supermarket, get more exercise by parking far away from the entrance rather than up close to the store. Start biking instead of driving. Walk your kids to school. When your children have a pool party, bring your bathing suit and swim. When your kids want to take their scooters out, try to run alongside them. Take a walk in the park or the woods.

Go to a farm and play with the animals. Take laps around the pond. Hike the trail at a local park. Have fun! Go to Bounce U or Sky Zone and jump around. It's great exercise, and you are moving your body.

Many people have started using standing desks at work. Look into it! Some companies might be amenable to helping pay for a Varidesk, which is a desk topper that can convert between sitting and standing heights. In standing at the office, you might even start a trend that will eventually benefit your work community, since everyone is standing and getting healthier and therefore using less sick days.

There are so many activities to try. Of course, sitting is comfortable, but it will have lasting negative impacts on your health that will be very uncomfortable later. If you HAVE to sit, make it a priority to get up every twenty minutes. But an even better alternative is to choose to do activities where you do not have to sit. Adjust your workplace and lifestyle to create more movement in your life, which will help you function better, feel better, and live better.

Chapter 14: Put the Pedal to the Metal

The most common heavy metal associated with memory problems and Alzheimer's disease is aluminum. Aluminum is found in most deodorants and antiperspirants. Besides containing aluminum, antiperspirants are also dangerous because they prevent sweating, which is very important for your health. It is one way our bodies manage the removal of waste and detoxify. When we put on antiperspirants, we clog up our sweat glands, thus restricting our armpits from sweating. It has been postulated that this can even lead to breast cancer. These products have metallic ingredients that can stay in our bodies and affect our brain health.

Aluminum is also found in the foil people use to store, pack, or cover food. This aluminum can seep into the foods we eat, where we directly ingest it. There may also be aluminum in the pans we use to cook food. There is aluminum in the cans that we use to store food. However, the good news is that there are easy solutions for all these problems. Instead of using aluminum, store your foods in glass containers. It is preferable to use stainless steel pans for cooking, which are safer than conventional pans. It is best to buy raw foods that are not stored in aluminum cans. These simple hints can help remove aluminum from your environment to help your brain perform at high levels, but we must avoid not only aluminum but all heavy metals and chemical toxins.

Another toxic chemical is mercury. Mercury poisoning is very common in America. The United States is one of the only countries that still allows mercury, in the form of Thimerosal, in flu vaccines. In my opinion, if you want to avoid the flu, you must build up your immune system. You must get proper rest, water, and sunlight. You must drink half your body weight in ounces per day. You must reduce stress, exercise, and eat healthily. You must get proper levels of vitamin D. In the winter, people get less vitamin D, drink less water, get less rest, go to more parties, stay out later, drink more alcohol, eat more food and desserts, exercise less, feel more unhappy, struggle with more financial pressure, and deal with more family stresses. These are the reasons people get the flu—not because they did not get a flu shot or because it is cold out. If you take care of your body, you won't get the flu! You won't need the shot, and you can avoid adding toxic mercury to your brain and body.

Mercury is also found in dental fillings. You should make sure that old fillings have been checked and are sealed properly. If there are any openings in the fillings, the mercury inside can leak into the bloodstream and eventually make it to your brain if you have inflammation. Therefore, it is imperative to remove these fillings before they cause irreversible damage. If, however, you have mercury fillings that are sealed properly, do not risk exposure by removing them when they are not causing any harm.

Fish is another common place mercury is found. The smaller the fish, the less mercury it has. Therefore, sardines, anchovies, and salmon are healthier choices. Also, it is important to buy fish from the Atlantic or the Mediterranean rather than the Pacific Ocean. The Pacific Ocean has a much higher percentage of radiated fish due to the accident at a Japanese nuclear plant that occurred as a result of a tsunami a few years ago.

It is not only the ocean that is filled with toxic chemicals and radioactive materials; our drinking water may contain toxic chemicals like fluoride or lead that may cause brain damage. Fluoride, the planet's most dangerous neurotoxin, is found in toothpaste as well, so I recommend getting fluoride-free toothpaste. Lead is also found in old paint and old houses in addition to our drinking water.

Think about where you might be encountering heavy metals and take steps to prevent continued exposure. Your brain health depends on being free from these harsh metals, and your health will benefit overall if you remove them from your life.

Chapter 15: A Breath of Fresh Air

To boost your brainpower, it is important to breathe correctly to get the proper amount of oxygen. The proper way to breath is a one-to-two ratio of inhale to exhale. If you inhale for two seconds, you must exhale for four seconds. Try to perform this, whenever you remember, for one week. The next week, extend your inhalation to three seconds and your exhalation to six seconds. Then the following week, inhale for four seconds and exhale for eight seconds. Repeat this process all the way up to inhaling for eight seconds and exhaling for sixteen seconds.

Breathe from your diaphragm. As you inhale, push your stomach down and out. Do not breathe from your shoulders or your chest. Look up slightly and bring back your shoulders as you breathe. To ensure you're getting enough oxygen, adding high-oxygen-producing plants in and around your household can help just as much as focusing on breathing. Three of the best oxygen-producing plants are snake plants, spider plants, and aloe vera. If you have yard space, I recommend planting trees there. One tree produces enough oxygen for five people.

When it comes to brain health, it is very important to monitor patients' oxygen levels. In our office, we use a pulse oximeter device. Most doctors believe that your blood oxygen percentage should be 95 percent and above, but as a functional neurologist, I recommend that it should be at 98 percent or higher. In addition to good nutrition and an active lifestyle, increasing oxygen levels through proper breathing and plant care is one of the most important factors in boosting your brainpower.

Chapter 16: Stop and Smell the Roses

S tress is extremely dangerous for your brain. In fact, your body responds to stress as if it were a disease. For this reason, it is healthy to do your absolute best to avoid stress. The three most significant stresses are physical stress, emotional stress, and biochemical stress. Physical stress could be from sitting at the computer all day and typing on the keyboard or using your phone. Emotional stress might result from being unsatisfied at work, being in a bad relationship, or having an unhealthy living situation. Biochemical stress can be due to toxins in our environment, like the pesticides in food, mercury in fish, fluoride in toothpaste, or aluminum in deodorant.

To combat the physical stresses, we must get the body moving. If you are sitting at the computer all day, make sure you participate in the 20 rule. Every twenty minutes, take a twenty-second break, walk twenty feet, and look twenty feet away. After a twenty-second break, you can go back to the computer. These activities will help prevent depression, back pain, headaches, heart disease, and Alzheimer's disease, along with improving the function of your brain and body. Another way to avoid physical stress is to make sure the body is balanced. For example, if you are playing golf and are always twisting in one direction, practice swinging the other way, so you don't just build the muscles on one side of your body. If you are a sanitation worker and are always tossing garbage over your left shoulder, start tossing it over your right shoulder. Make sure you do not do activities that only use one part of your body. This will avoid physical imbalances and help your brain and body function better and feel better.

Emotional stress is even more important to deal with than the physical. To do so, you might have to move out of a big city and into the suburbs, to seek out nature and relative calm. Or you might have to quit an unsatisfying job. Maybe one that pays well, but where the hours add stress to your life, where your boss is mean, and where you don't get along with your coworkers. In this case, the stress is not worth the money. Without your health, nothing else matters, including money.

Emotional stress is a true "silent killer." Monday morning is the most common time for a heart attack. People are stressed out about going to a job they hate. The worst phrase in the world is, "Thank God it's Friday." It means that people hate their life and can't wait for the weekend. You should love to wake up Monday morning—full of energy and excited to go to work. Your job should be rewarding and related to your passion. It should involve helping others and allow room for growth and progress. Progress is vital to boost your brainpower.

The brain needs progress to grow and reduce emotional stress. The more your brain progresses, the better it functions. If you truly want to boost your brainpower, you must progress in all aspects of life.

You must progress in your personal relationships, always looking for ways to improve them. Remember, everyone's needs are different. You might be in a relationship where your spouse likes to be heard. In that case, progress is working on listening more. Other people love to be acknowledged, so progress would be acknowledging their spouses more frequently. Some people like physical affection, others like gifts, some like quality time, others like to be complimented, some people like gratitude, and others like space. The point is that everyone is different, and their needs might be different than your needs. Making progress in relationships requires paying attention to and empathizing with their needs.

In addition to your personal relationships, it is important to progress in your health. This means working on all the health tips in the previous chapters. A great way to monitor your progress is through blood work.

You must also make progress in your job or career to reduce emotional stress. Climb the ladder to success. Keep on increasing your income and increasing your charity. Help more people. Give bigger tips. Give people more compliments. Thank people more. Have more gratitude. Pray more. Meditate deeper. Be more mindful. Improve your physical and mental fitness. Eat healthier. Get a more restful sleep. Love more people. Bring more joy. Have more fun. Tell more jokes. Smile more frequently. Learn more. Teach more. Listen more. Talk less. Worry less. Complain less. Think less. Stress less. Fight less. Hold fewer grudges. Gossip less. Stop reading and watching the news. Watch less TV and Netflix. Use social media less. Use your cell phone less. Check your email less. Spend more time with people. If you spend more time outside and in nature, this will decrease your emotional stress.

The third major type of stress is biochemical stress. This includes the chemicals we are exposed to in our lives. In Chapter 3, we discussed many products that contain chemicals we should avoid, like aerosol sprays, deodorants, bleaches, perfumes, Febreeze, Lysol, colognes, and most suntan lotions. These products are not only toxic to the environment, but they are also toxic to inhale and are toxic to your skin.

If you reduce the three stresses mentioned in this chapter, you are less likely to be affected by the most common chronic conditions and will therefore function better, feel better, and live better.

Chapter 17: Blood is Thicker than Water

If you want to be healthy and develop strong brain function, it is important to make sure your blood work is done regularly and that your levels are in the "healthy" range. Keep in mind that I'm talking about the healthy range, not the "normal" range. When you get blood work done, and the doctor or the lab tells you that it's normal, they are saying that your ranges are normal compared to an average patient's blood work. Remember that most Americans are living an unhealthy lifestyle with a poor diet, lack of exercise, high stress, high alcohol consumption, limited sleep, and lack of hydration. So, if you are "normal," you are like a typical unhealthy American.

As a result, in my office, we have created a healthy range for all our blood tests where you are compared to people living a very healthy lifestyle. If your blood work is in this healthy range, then you are less likely to develop heart disease, diabetes, cancer, or dementia. Blood work can also discover any nutritional deficiencies. Many patients take vitamins or supplements that are extremely dangerous and can affect your brain and gut function negatively. Just because it is a "natural" supplement does not mean it is not dangerous. Earlier in the book, I mentioned how medication can be dangerous, but be aware that taking vitamins can be dangerous as well. For example, I have a sixty-year-old female patient who we'll call Amy. She told me that she was taking calcium supplements every day for the past ten years. I asked her why, and she responded that her doctor told her it was good for her bones. Calcium supplements are very dangerous. These supplements have been linked to cancer, heart disease, arthritis, and brain dysfunction.

In my opinion, you should only take calcium supplements if you are deficient in calcium, not because it is good for your bones or because you have osteoporosis. Do not take B12 for energy or because you are a vegetarian. Do not take magnesium to help with digestion or sleep. Do not take iron because you think you are anemic. Only take vitamins if your lab results show that you are deficient in a particular vitamin or mineral. The most common deficiency I see is vitamin D—I have had low levels myself and therefore take high-quality vitamin D that must be ordered by a doctor. Please remember that many supplements can be dangerous, so it is vital to check your blood work before taking any. Monitoring your blood work is a crucial step to staying healthy and preventing serious neurological disorders.

Chapter 18: All's Well that Ends Well

It's true; there is no magic pill for brain health. For most American people, it requires commitment to several lifestyle changes. This approach to brain health starts with YOU— your conscious choices about the types of foods you eat, the quality of the water you drink, the products you use on your body, and the exercise you get. I acknowledge that the information in this book might seem overwhelming at first. Many of these changes require some planning and patience while you form new and better habits. Trying to change all at once is an enormous commitment for most people, and it's definitely not always easy. But as you adapt to new ways of living, these new habits will eventually become second nature, and you will find happiness in experiencing the lasting benefits of health.

If you read this book and are anxious about how many years you have been eating a certain diet or using certain products, I encourage you to remember this: *it is never too late to make changes for your health*. Although things like chemicals on non-stick pans could eventually lead to health problems, that does not mean all hope is lost if you have been cooking with them for many years. Remember, the human body is very strong and adaptable. However, today is the best day to make changes to your life for your health, not tomorrow.

Try to really meditate on your daily life and habits. If there are activities you do or foods you eat every day, it is important to consider whether these things are serving you and your health. If you have been stressed and unhappy at the same job for years, today might be the day to start looking at help wanted ads. If you're fed up with being exhausted after going up flights of stairs, perhaps tonight is the night you go for your first long walk in the park. Or maybe stop by the produce section of your local grocery store instead of a drive-through restaurant on your way home from work. Sometimes changes are unnerving; there is no doubt about that. But believe me, you are more than capable of change, and once you start, getting healthy is exciting and empowering.

Don't do it alone. If you have a family member who has been enacting new healthy diets, jump on the bandwagon! Everyone involved will benefit. If there are people in your life who have expressed a desire to change their lives, be the catalyst. Let your hope for better health be the seed of a community. Start a walking or hiking group! Get together with a group of friends and neighbors for a healthy potluck dinner every week. When you think about healthy living, don't imagine eating broccoli sad and alone. Think of new friends and activities, great exercise, a long life with your loved ones, and a better quality of life. This is the joy that comes with changing your life today.

I believe people should have a team of healthcare providers and wellness-oriented people in their corner. After you have started with functional neurology and applied neuroscience, you can also try acupuncture, massage therapy, Reiki, yoga, personal training, or nutritional therapy. There are so many brilliant practitioners who can enrich your life and keep your health on track. You owe it to yourself to explore your options. Finding the right practitioner can be a game-changer, especially for people struggling with autoimmune diseases, complex disorders, or chronic pain.

I truly hope that you will take this opportunity to rewire your brain with these techniques. I have seen thousands of lives turn around through the implementation of techniques I learned at the Carrick Institute and in studying neuroscience. It is a misconception that neurology is only about the brain and nervous system. The brain controls every part of the body. From digestion and metabolism to the function of your heart; the brain does more than cognition. When we treat the brain, we treat the whole body. That is why functional neurology and neuroplasticity are so powerful.

I hope you have learned a lot from these pages, but understand that this is not the end—it's just the beginning. The only thing you have to do is make the choice. Choose to be happy. Choose to be healthy. Choose to love. Choose to give.

Remember, the best day to plant a tree was ten years ago. The next best day is today. As they say: a journey of a thousand miles begins with the first step. Let's make that first step together today.

References, Breakthroughs, and Further Reading:

The following is a list of neuroscientific studies relating to or involving memory and brain function. Information in these articles has served as inspiration in my work and has helped many people struggling with memory loss and countless other neurological problems.

This is by no means an exhaustive list of the research in this field, which is vast. But this may be a starting point for you. I hope that you will find these sources useful in your own research into the health of your brain.

AUTOIMMUNE CONDITIONS

Microglia in neurodegenerative disease.
Perry VH1, Nicoll JA, Holmes C.Nat Rev Neurol. 2010 Apr;6(4): 193-201. doi:10.1038/nrneurol.2010.17. Epub 2010 Mar 16.

Oxidative stress, mitochondrial damage and neurodegenerative diseases.
Guo C1, Sun L2, Chen X3, Zhang D4.Neural Regen Res. 2013 Jul 25;8(21):2003-14. doi:10.3969/j.issn.1673-5374.2013.21.009.

Systemic inflammatory cells fight off neurodegenerative disease.
Schwartz M1, Shechter R.Nat Rev Neurol. 2010 Jul;6(7):405-10. doi: 10.1038/nrneurol.2010.71. Epub 2010 Jun 8.

Systemic immune challenges trigger and drive Alzheimer-like neuropathology in mice
Krstic D1, Madhusudan A, Doehner J, Vogel P, Notter T, Imhof C, Manalastas A, Hilfiker M, Pfister S, Schwerdel C, Riether C, Meyer U, Knuesel I. J Neuroinflammation. 2012 Jul 2;9:151.

doi: 10.1186/1742-2094-9-151.

CHEMICAL EXPOSURE

Environmental pollutants as risk factors for neurodegenerative disorders: Alzheimer and Parkinson diseases.

Chin-Chan M1, Navarro-Yepes J1, Quintanilla-Vega B1.
Front Cell Neurosci. 2015 Apr 10;9:124. doi:10.3389/fncel.2015.00124. eCollection 2015.

DIET

Alzheimer's disease and epigenetic diet.

Sezgin Z1, Dincer Y2. Neurochem Int. 2014 Dec;78:105-16. doi: 10.1016/j.neuint.2014.09.012. Epub 2014 Oct 5.

How does diabetes accelerate Alzheimer's disease pathology?

Sims-Robinson C1, Kim B, Rosko A, Feldman EL.
Nat Rev Neurol. 2010 Oct;6(10):551-9. doi: 10.1038/nrneurol.2010.130. Epub 2010 Sep 14.

Intermittent fasting protects against Alzheimer's disease, possibly through restoring Aquaporin-4 polarity.

Jingzhu Zhang,1,† Zhipeng Zhan,1,2,† Xinhui Li,1 Aiping Xing,1 Congmin Jiang,1 Yanqiu Chen,1 Wanying Shi,3,* andLi An1,*
Front Mol Neurosci. 2017; 10: 395.

Ketogenic diet in neuromuscular and neurodegenerative diseases.

Paoli A1, Bianco A2, Damiani E1, Bosco G1. Biomed Res Int. 2014;2014:474296. doi: 10.1155/2014/474296. Epub 2014 Jul

Neuroprotective action of omega-3 polyunsaturated fatty acids against neurodegenerative diseases: evidence from

animal studies.

Calon F1, Cole G. Prostaglandins Leukot Essent Fatty Acids. 2007 Nov-Dec;77(5-6):287-93. Epub 2007 Nov 26.

The emerging role of nutrition in Parkinson's disease
Stacey E. Seidl,1,† Jose A. Santiago,1,† Hope Bilyk,2 and Judith A. Potashkin1,* Front Aging Neurosci. 2014; 6: 36.

FUNCTIONAL NEUROLOGY

The effectiveness of neurofeedback on cognitive functioning in patients with Alzheimer's disease: Preliminary results.

Luijmes RE, et al. Neurophysiol Clin. 2016. Neurophysiol Clin. 2016 Jun;46(3):179-87. doi: 10.1016/j.neucli.2016.05.069. Epub 2016 Jun 30.

EYES

Antisaccade task reflects cortical involvement in mild cognitive impairment.

Heuer HW1, Mirsky JB, Kong EL, Dickerson BC, Miller BL, Kramer JH, Boxer AL. Neurology. 2013 Oct 1;81(14):1235-43. doi: 10.1212/WNL.0b013e3182a6cbfe. Epub 2013 Aug 28.

Eye movement alterations during reading in patients with early Alzheimer's disease.

Fernández G1, Mandolesi P, Rotstein NP, Colombo O, Agamennoni O, Politi LE. Invest Ophthalmol Vis Sci. 2013 Dec 30;54(13):8345-52. doi: 10.1167/iovs.13-12877.

Saccade abnormalities in autopsy-confirmed frontotemporal lobar degeneration and Alzheimer disease.

Boxer AL1, Garbutt S, Seeley WW, Jafari A, Heuer HW, Mirsky J, Hellmuth J, Trojanowski JQ, Huang E, DeArmond S, Neuhaus J, Miller BL. Arch Neurol. 2012 Apr;69(4):509-17. doi:

10.1001/archneurol.2011.1021.

VITAMINS

Vitamin D deficiency and Alzheimer's disease: Common links.
Keeney JT1, Butterfield DA2 Neurobiol Dis. 2015 Dec;84:84-98. doi: 10.1016/j.nbd.2015.06.020. Epub 2015 Jul 6.

Made in the USA
Middletown, DE
19 November 2021